Distribution, publication, and copying in any form are prohibited and subject to damages.

TEN HYPNOSES

Copying, publishing, and sharing with third parties are only permitted with the written consent of the author. Please observe the notes on copyright and usage.

Distribution, publication, and copying in any form are prohibited and subject to damages.

Copying, publishing, and sharing with third parties are only permitted with the written consent of the author. Please observe the notes on copyright and usage.

Distribution, publication, and copying in any form are prohibited and subject to damages.

Ingo Michael Simon

TEN HYPNOSES

7

PSYCHO-ONCOLOGY

Copying, publishing, and sharing with third parties are only permitted with the written consent of the author. Please observe the notes on copyright and usage.

Distribution, publication, and copying in any form are prohibited and subject to damages.

© 2024 Ingo Michael Simon
All rights reserved.
Independently published
www.ingosimon.com

Important Notes for Urgent Attention:
The contents of this book are based on the practical experiences of the author with hypnosis applications and psychotherapy in a trance state. Although the author has strived for the utmost care, errors or misunderstandings in the presentation cannot be completely excluded. Therapeutic work with people and the application of hypnosis are solely the responsibility of the hypnotist. It cannot be ruled out that parts of this book may be misunderstood or that the application of a presented procedure may cause an undesirable reaction in the client. The author also assumes no co-responsibility if work with a client is carried out with reference to the statements in this book.

The Author:
Ingo Michael Simon studied psychology and education and is a hypnotherapist with practices in southwestern Germany and Switzerland. With the help of hypnosis-supported psychotherapy, he primarily treats people with persistent psychological conditions. His practice focuses on anxiety disorders, pathological compulsions, and psychosomatic illnesses. His therapeutic offerings mainly include classical and modern hypnosis applications and the dreamland therapy he developed himself.

Copying, publishing, and sharing with third parties are only permitted with the written consent of the author. Please observe the notes on copyright and usage.

Distribution, publication, and copying in any form are prohibited and subject to damages.

Notes on Copyright and Usage

Copying, publishing, and sharing with third parties is prohibited and only permitted with the written consent of the author. Please observe the following copyright and usage guidelines.

This work has been carefully crafted and created to the best of the author's knowledge and personal experience. It comprises text templates and application guidelines for professional hypnosis sessions. The author is a licensed psychotherapist with extensive experience in psychotherapy, coaching, and personal training using hypnotic techniques and methods. Nevertheless, the author and the publisher assume no liability for the accuracy of information, instructions, and advice, nor for any typographical errors. The author and publisher accept no responsibility or liability for the application of these texts and recommendations with clients or patients, nor for any potential consequences or unexpected reactions. It is expressly noted that the application of therapeutic and advisory techniques and formulations lies solely and entirely within the responsibility of the practitioner. This also applies to adherence to the boundaries of legally regulated medical and therapeutic practices. The fact that a book containing action proposals is freely available for sale does not imply that its application with clients or patients is permitted for everyone.

Copying, publishing, and sharing with third parties are only permitted with the written consent of the author. Please observe the notes on copyright and usage.

Distribution, publication, and copying in any form are prohibited and subject to damages.

Copying, publishing, and sharing with third parties are only permitted with the written consent of the author. Please observe the notes on copyright and usage.

Distribution, publication, and copying in any form are prohibited and subject to damages.

Table of contents

Introduction 9
#1 11
#2 16
#3 21
#4 27
#5 33
#6 38
#7 43
#8 48
#9 53
#10 58
Overview of All Titles in the Series "Ten Hypnoses" 63

Copying, publishing, and sharing with third parties are only permitted with the written consent of the author. Please observe the notes on copyright and usage.

Distribution, publication, and copying in any form are prohibited and subject to damages.

Copying, publishing, and sharing with third parties are only permitted with the written consent of the author. Please observe the notes on copyright and usage.

Introduction

The series "Ten Hypnoses" is very well known in Germany, Austria, and Switzerland as a collection of texts for therapeutic work and is used by numerous psychotherapeutic practices, doctors, therapists, coaches, and other helping professionals. I am pleased to now be able to offer these texts in other countries as well.

Most therapists have their own methods for inducing and deepening trance as well as for exiting trance. Therefore, I have focused on the main part of the hypnosis. The texts in this book can be integrated as the main part into any hypnosis process.

The texts in this collection use various hypnosis techniques. I will not explain these in detail, as I assume that users have the appropriate training. It is also not necessary to understand the exact structure or functioning of the different parts. The texts can simply be read aloud, and they will have their effect.

Decide for yourself which text best suits your client or patient at any given time. You can also combine passages from different texts. It is not about using all ten hypnoses in sequence. It is a selection of possibilities.

I want to emphasize that books cannot replace therapy. Psychotherapy or other therapeutic treatments involve much more. A careful diagnosis is the necessary basis for deciding on the use of methods, including whether hypnosis or one of my texts should be used. Even in this case, preparatory discussions, follow-up discussions during the session, and of course, a therapeutic concept for the sequence of sessions and the content approaches are essential parts of therapy. This cannot and should not be achieved with a collection of texts.

In any case, I wish you much success in your work and I am pleased if my text templates can contribute in a small way.

Ingo Michael Simon

#1

For Those Affected

... ... You often feel physically tired and burned out ... ... powerless and drained ... ... you feel how chemotherapy affects the body, causes nausea and exhaustion ... ... maybe even pain sometimes ... ... but you know that the treatment will help you ... ... you have yourself therefore made to see it through ... ... and it is really quite remarkable how much courage and strength you have already mustered to actually go through it all ... ... Now it comes down to it to find peace and relaxation again so that your body can recover from the strenuous treatment ... ...let your breathing become conscious and breathe in and out consciously ... ... very consciously ... ... in ... ...and off ... ... [in the actual breathing rhythm of the client please] ... ... on ... ... and off ... ... if you once paying attention to your breath, you can clearly feel the air coming in and out through your nose flows out ... ... with every breath ... ... you can feel it ... ... through breathing you can body now find rest ... ... To do this, imagine that you are in your entire body could breathe into it ... ... as if fresh air flows through your whole body with every breath flows ... ... and when you breathe out it relaxes even more and becomes calmer ... ... Let's start with your arms ... ... Breathe in deeply and feel the air flowing into your arms ... ... very deep ... ... down to the fingertips ... ... and when you breathe out, the air flows back again ... ...if there was still tension now, you could feel it because the air wouldn't flow unhindered ... ... so if there is something left, you can let go of it with the exhale ...... And your arms become calmer ... This is how you do it with the next breaths ... ... your arms relax more and more ... ... the left arm ... ... and also the right arm ... ... Now to the head ... ... Pay attention to your breath and direct it to the head ... ... You can feel how the breath pulls through the nose to behind the eyes ... ... The fresh air is distributed in your whole head ... ... You can let go of everything that is disturbing you with the exhalation and afterwards lead outside...... thoughts or considerations...... doubts or fears...... With every breath your head relaxes...... deeper and deeper...... so your head becomes whole free and carefree ... ... completely free and calm ... ... with the next breaths, the air flows into your upper body ... ... first into the lungs ... ... and from there on into the muscles of the back and abdomen ... ... into all internal organs ... ... Here, too, you would notice if there were obstacles ... ... if something was still tense should be, then you feel it and can dissolve it ... ... and when you breathe out you let go of it ... ...your upper body comes to rest ... ... You allow your upper body to experience rest ... ...as you continue to breathe in peace, your body relaxes more and more ... ... all parts of your body, which have already been mentioned, deepen the rest and relaxation ... ... with every breath ... ... with every single breath ... ...you're doing well ... ... It's just as right as you are doing it right now ... ... So your relaxes your body best and comes to new strength and strength ... ... And if you have forgotten something or have overlooked something ... ... then you can do it now in move your legs ... ... with a few breaths your whole upper body fills ... ... also your arms and your head with oxygen ... ... and when you breathe out any tension that might be gone has remained here and there, in your legs ... ... Now everything that could still be disturbing flows into yours legs............ You breathe in deeply, and the air flows very deep into your legs...... You breathe out and everything that somehow disturbs or pinches ... ... everything that is now still tense or cramped flows while over the soles of your feet to the outside ... ... With each exhalation you let go of tension and send them out over the soles of your feet and the tips of your toes ... ... and you'll be there calmer ... ... and your body comes to rest and relaxes completely ... ... more and more ... ... and more and more ... ... Well, it's exactly right ... ... You are doing the right thing, and it's very simple ... ... You just have to breathe in and out, that's enough ... ... [in the rhythm of the client please] ... ... on and off ... ... that's enough ... ... on and off ... ... that's enough ... ...now you can enjoy the relaxation...... You feel how relaxed your body feels...... maybe as relaxed as it has not been for a long time...... And maybe are you asking yourself if you can give your body even more rest ... ... if it is possible, right now to relax even deeper now and give your body some rest ... ... Then you just breathe more ... ... Every breath helps you ... ... Every breath gently caresses your body ... ... Now you will surely also feel how good it is when you create this calm state for your body ... ... how relaxing it is ... ... you feel it more and more clearly and at the same time see how simply it is ... ... your body finds strength and courage again ... ... hope and strength ... ... balance and healing power ... ... new healing power ... ...

... ... But every day your body can and may recover ... ... regenerate from all the stresses ... ... You can help him, just like today ...... just like now .... You just make yourself comfortable every day for a while ...... as comfortable as you can, also and especially then, if you are feeling sick or in pain ...... You find a while every day of peace, ... and your breathing will help you find peace and calm even deeper and your body to purify ...... to find new strength ...... new freshness ...... vitality and strength ...... exactly like that like now and maybe even more ...... because your deep inside learns better every time, how it can take the path of rest and renewal ... your deep inside learns with each time better how it can help you regenerate your body ...... help it get healthy ... ...

#2

For Relatives

... ... Chemotherapy is exhausting and dangerous treatment ... ... But it is not only then Stress, if you were affected by it yourself ... ... You know what it is like to accompany a loved one in getting through chemotherapy ... ... That's a stress for you too ... ... because you are worried about how things will continue ... ... because you don't have the disease yourself can influence and sometimes have the feeling of having to watch helplessly and wait ... ... Then you have a lot of thoughts ... ... So you also need a way to come to terms with all this, to become lighter and to let go of burdens again and again ... ... You too want to be healthy and stay healthy ... ... and you have every right in this world to do so ... ...Today you can concentrate completely on yourself...... Today it should only be about you and your health is going ... ... Maybe you think that you are already healthy ... ... Yes Health is more than the absence of illness ... ... health means joy of life ... ... Strength ... ... hope ... ... you can be healthy and feel good ... ... so you start with to allow yourself to feel good ... ... even and especially if it is a loved one If things go bad, you have to be allowed to feel good, because only healthy and strong can you muster the strength to help him / her ... ... It's really amazing how well you are doing at this moment, you to allow yourself to be healthy once ... ... with a clear conscience ... ... This is exactly what you concentrate more and more on ... ... on your good conscience, because that is exactly what you are entitled to ... ...Allow yourself once again very clearly to be healthy and even more, to feel good ... ... you can feel good ... ... Enjoy this moment in which you can feel really good ... ... right now ... ... right here ... ... exactly like this ... ... If you listen deeply into yourself, you will feel that you have become tired yourself...... that yours Body sends signals of exhaustion...... So next you concentrate on your body feeling ... ... Today you allow your body to relax very intensely...... to rest and in the process to come to new strength ... ... It is remarkable how well you manage your body to send this signal ... ... to allow your body to finally come to rest now ... ... because that's exactly what helps you to stay healthy ... ... stronger and more self-confident ... ... and with it Much healthier ... ... The more you manage to be and stay healthy yourself, the better can you actually do for your sick relatives ... ... [Please add here who it is acts ... for your sick mother ... ...] ... ... to be there ... ... always give yourself and your body a gift more mindfulness and love ... ... mindfulness and love ... ... just like that ... ... With every breath your mindfulness becomes more intense ... ... the mindfulness of you for you ... ... more intensely with every single breath ... ... So pay close attention to your breath and let it go to flow very consciously ... ... Follow the pull of your breath and show your body that you are Allowing him rest and health ... ... It is great how well you manage to help yourself and your body to finally come to rest and find new strength ... ... new health for you ... ... because that's exactly what you deserve ... ... Breathe calmly and evenly ... ... just like that ... just like that ... ... Then you deal with your feelings of guilt ... ... You often have this strange one Feeling that healthy people often have when a relative gets sick ... ... the healthy ones People then feel uncomfortable and secretly guilty because they are allowed to be healthy themselves ... ... But this thinking is a mistake ... ... We can all get healthy ... ... be healthy ... ... and stay healthy ... ... we have good wishes for our sick ... ... prayers and hopes ...

...We don't know when they can be healthy again ... ... But you can be healthy with a clear conscience ... ... healthy with a clear conscience ... ... now in this calm ... ... here and today ...... at this very moment you can see it that way ... ... you can see that you are innocent ... ... you can now let go of your feelings of guilt ... ... You can do just that now ... ... you let go of all negative thoughts ... ... you let go of every bad conscience ... ... you let go of everyone Feel free to guilt ... ... because that's the way it is ... ... that's how it should be ... ... free from guilt and healthy ... ... and with every breath the feeling of inner freedom becomes bigger and clearer ... ... with every single breath it becomes clearer to you and this thought becomes more stable: I am innocent ... ... I am innocent ... ... With every breath you can hear it deep inside you like your own voice ... ... I am innocent ... ... I am innocent ... ... With every breath the feeling of inner freedom more intense ... ... freedom from all guilt ... ... with every single breath more intensely ... ... So pay close attention to your breath and let it flow very consciously ... ... Follow that Take your breath and hear your inner voice that says: I am innocent ... ... Yes, I am and remain without guilt ... ... I am free...... I am free...... It is remarkable how well you manage to hear your inner voice and to accept its words ... ... Very remarkable, how good you are now can help yourself by being important to yourself and taking care of yourself ... ... you today and keep thinking about your self-awareness ... ...

... ... My words and the words of your inner voice are deeply anchored in your subconscious ... ...Everything is deeply impressed in your feelings ... ... So you can every day, if you want, breathe in a very targeted way for letting go and breathe for your inner freedom ... ... Whenever you are completely Breathe out consciously and deliberately slowly and for a long time, because you want to let go, you immediately feel the inner one Liberation ... ... becoming lighter ... ... you simply exhale slowly and long in a targeted manner and feel your letting go ... ... Whenever you have the feeling that old thoughts might come back, you just breathe out slowly and long ... ... slowly and long ... ... and let go let's go ... ... just like today ... ... just like today ... ... In this way you will always find strength to support your loved ones ... ... [please insert the person being looked after or affected] ... ... to continue his recovery accompany ... ...

continue to bear the stresses of chemo together with him / her ... ...

#3

For Those Affected

The following hypnosis session works with a symbolic anchor. One calls an anchor a trigger that can create a certain feeling or arouse a certain thought should. We want to help the client, by holding a hand flatterer, the feeling of a strong self-healing power in the form of great trust in one's own deep-seated powers to call consciousness. To do this, it is necessary to first establish a state in which the Client in trance consciously experiences self-confidence and positive thoughts. This feeling will then associated and anchored with the grasping and holding of a hand flatterer. Subsequently in phases of despair and discouragement, the client should be able to use this hand flatterer as an aid to get back into a state of hope and despair as quickly as possible Trust to arrive. Any hand flatterer that the client likes or agrees with can be used, also a healing stone. It always depends on the balance between realistic healing prospects and forward-looking thoughts of healing Find. On the one hand, hope and belief in healing should be more optimistic than the prognosis, in order to really get to the self-healing potential of the organism that not is accessible to the mind. On the other hand, the gap between suggestion and imaginable healing should not become implausible; otherwise the effect of hypnosis is quickly lost. To put it very directly: Although there are also "miraculous healings", it makes no sense in hypnotized to claim that stray cancer will soon go away if only the thoughts are positive enough. Overall, psychotherapeutic treatment of cancer is primarily about dealing with the disease and the changes it is having in the client's life brings himself to deal with. This is more important than healing suggestions. At the same time, my experience shows that believers in self-healing powers and deep-seated energies of the organism often makes an essential contribution to recovery, both for the inner attitude towards the treatment and recovery process as well as for the actual question of the healing prospects. With this, as with all hypnoses in the book, please note that there is always an individual adjustment to the specific illness and condition of the client.

... ... I will now help you to really activate your own self-healing power ... ... it can help you to make as clear progress as possible in recovery ... ... What we call self-healing power can also help you to get through difficult phases of treatment more easily, to find hope and trust again and again ... ...strength for the next Steps ... ...To this end, today we will jointly strengthen the self-healing power of your organism .... But first you can make yourself really comfortable, now find peace ... ... you will. Inwardly more and more calm and concentrate only on the feeling of calm ... ... After all the stresses and strains, you now deserve rest ... ... Sink deeper and deeper into a wonderful trance ... ... deeper and deeper ... ... with every word that I say you go a little deeper in this beautiful state of inner calm ... ... you're doing it right, you just allow it, just let it happen and drift all by yourself, at your own pace, at your own pace in this beautiful state of deep ... ... inner ... ... calm ... ... good so ... ... very good ......Now feel deep inside you the trust in yourself ... ... Your deep trust is waiting deep inside you and can get stronger ... ... sink deeper and deeper and find your trust in yourself ... ... so You have already experienced and endured a lot, because only your trust in you and your strength has this enables you ... ... the more you manage to get into a calm state, the more you feel this trust ... ... and you are already in a calm state, so you have already found the trust ... ... maybe without noticing it, but it is here ... ... deep in you ... ... let this trust become more and more evident, because you need it now ... ... it is here ...... deep inside you ... ... let this trust become even stronger, because you need it now ... ... itis here ... ... deep within you ... ... you have found it ... ... excellent ... ... because if you have found it, and you have, then it becomes clearer at precisely this moment ... ... at this very moment ... ... good so ... ... very, very good so ... ...It is this inner trust that helps you ... ... It helps you get through difficult times ... It helps you to be strong and to recover quickly ... ... It helps you to have the greatest possible strength in you awaken and use ... ... your inner self-healing power ... ... the power of your organism, yourself to heal yourself as well and as far as possible lies in precisely this inner trust ... ... you can use it very particularly today, because now she is in a state of inner calm, in a trance more freely and can move unhindered ... ... Now your organism helps you to heal your Illness particularly intense ... ... The more you trust yourself or simply if you concentrate on the idea of trust, the more your organism can now help with healing ... ...I will now give you the flatterer in the hand ... ... [Name the symbol actually used ... the healing stone... the wooden lion etc.] ... ... take it and hold it tight ... ... it should be your healing anchor ... ...that's right ... ... Hold on to your healing anchor and at the same time feel the trust deep within you...... Both become one...... your healing anchor and your trust...... This is how both work together...... Because whenever you feel your healing anchor in your hand, it immediately becomes your deep one trust awake and help you with all your inner power of self-healing ... ... now and every time, when you take the healing anchor in your hand, you feel your inner trust very strongly ... ... like now, even more clearly ... ...

... ... Hold the healing anchor tight now ... ... Concentrate on the feeling in your hand ... ... this feeling shows you now and in the future that your organism has all the power to heal itself ... ... You will feel even more trust and confidence ... ... every day you can activate and strengthen this trust and also the power of healing by taking the healing anchor, your personal healing anchor, in your hand and feeling it with your eyes closed ...... You can move it in your hand, feel it…… or you can hold it and press it… … do it the way it feels best … … just take your healing anchor every day in your hand and feel it and your organism immediately provides trust and healing power … … trust and healing power … … just like now … … just like now … … hold your healing anchor firmly so that it connects even more with you … … with your healing power … …

… … [Continue the transition and let the client hold the healing anchor until hold the end of the session.] … …

#4

For Relatives

The following hypnosis session works with a symbolic anchor. One calls an anchor a trigger that can create a certain feeling or arouse a certain thought should. We want to help the client, by holding a hand flatterer, the feeling of a strong self-healing power in the form of great trust in one's own deep-seated powers to call consciousness. To do this, it is necessary to first establish a state in which the Client in trance consciously experiences self-confidence and positive thoughts. This feeling will then associated and anchored with the grasping and holding of a hand flatterer. Subsequently in phases of despair and discouragement, the client should be able to use this hand flatterer as an aid to get back into a state of hope and despair as quickly as possible Trust to arrive. Any hand flatterer that the client likes or agrees with can be used, also a healing stone. It always depends on the balance between realistic healing prospects and forward-looking thoughts of healing Find. On the one hand, hope and belief in healing should be more optimistic than the prognosis, in order to really get to the self-healing potential of the organism that not is accessible to the mind. On the other hand, the gap between suggestion and imaginable healing should not become implausible; otherwise the effect of hypnosis is quickly lost. To put it very directly: Although there are also "miraculous healings", it makes no sense in hypnotized to claim that stray cancer will soon go away if only the thoughts are positive enough. Overall, psychotherapeutic treatment of cancer is primarily about dealing with the disease and the changes it is having in the client's life brings himself to deal with. This is more important than healing suggestions. At the same time, my experience shows that believers in self-healing powers and deep-seated energies of the organism often makes an essential contribution to recovery, both for the inner attitude towards the treatment and recovery process as well as for the actual question of the healing prospects. With this, as with all hypnoses in the book, please note that there is always an individual adjustment to the specific illness and condition of the client.

… … I will now help you to really activate your own self-healing power … … it can help you to regain a balanced mental state in order to be healthy stay … … and if you feel sick or attacked yourself, maybe exhausted and drained, then your inner strength will help you to become completely healthy and strong again … …what we call self-healing power can also help you through difficult phases of treatment of your dear relatives … … [better name … your son … your father etc.] … … easier to get through, to find hope and trust again and again … … strength for the next steps … … Today we will strengthen the self-healing power of your organism together … …First, however, you can make yourself really comfortable, now find peace … … You become more and calmer inside and only concentrate on the feeling of calm … … After all the stresses and strains and effort you deserve rest now…… Sink deeper and deeper into a wonderful trance…… Deeper and deeper…… with every word I say, you go a little deeper into this wonderful state of inner calm…… You are doing it right, you just let it happen, you just let it happen and drive all by itself, at your speed, at your own pace in these beautiful state of deep … … inner … … calm … … good so … … very good … …Now feel deep inside you the trust in yourself ... ... Your deep trust is waiting deep inside you and can get stronger ... ... sink deeper and deeper and find your trust in yourself ... ... so you have already experienced and endured a lot, because only your trust in you and your strength has this enables you ... ... you know many difficult phases in your own life ... ... maybe also serious illnesses ... ... and also the accompaniment of your loved one ... ... [better concrete name ... your son ... your father etc.] ... ... is a difficult time for you, in which you too have strength have left and can use help ... ... The more you manage to get into a calm state, the more you will feel this too trust in you that can help you to get through all of this ... ... and be in a calm state you do, so you've already found confidence ... ... maybe without noticing it, but it is here ... ... deep within you ... ... let this trust become clearer and clearer, because you need it now ... ... it is here ... ... deep within you ... ... let this trust become even stronger, because you need it now ... ... it is here ... ... deep inside you ... ... you found it ... ... out outstanding ... ... because when you have found it, and you have it, then it will be exactly in this one Moment clearer ... ... exactly at this moment ... ... good that way ...

... very, very good that way ... ... It is this inner trust that helps you ... ... It helps you get through difficult times ... It helps you to be strong and to recover quickly ... ... It helps you to have the greatest possible strength in you awaken and use ... ... your inner self-healing power ... ... the power of your organism, yourself Balancing or healing yourself as well and as much as possible over and over again is exactly what you need this inner trust ... ... You can use it very particularly today, because now in the state of inner peace, in a trance, she is freer and can move unhindered ... ... Now yours will help you Organism is particularly intense in healing your illness ... ... The more you focus on that Trust or just focus on the idea of trust, all the more it can help your organism to heal now ... ... I will now give you the flatterer in the hand ... ... [Name the symbol actually used ... the healing stone ... the wooden lion etc.] ... ... take it and hold it tight ... ... it should be your anchor of strength ... ... That's right ... ... hold on to your power anchor and at the same time feel the trust deep inside you ... ... Both become one ... ... your anchor of strength and your trust ... ... This is how both work together...... Because whenever you feel your power anchor in your hand, your deep trust immediately becomes awake and helps you with all your inner power of self-healing ... ... now and every time you take the healing anchor in your hand, you feel your inner trust very strongly ... ... like now, even more clearly ... ...

... ... Hold the power anchor tight now ... ... Concentrate on the feeling in your hand ... ... this feeling shows you now and in the future that your organism has all the power to heal itself ... ... So you feel even more trust and confidence ... ... Every day you can activate and strengthen this trust and also the power of healing by using the power anchor, take your personal power anchor in your hand and feel it with your eyes closed ... ... You can move it in your hand, feel it ... ... or you can hold it and press it ... ... Do it the way it feels best ... ... just put your power anchor in your hand every Hand and feel it and immediately your organism provides trust and healing power ... ... trust and healing power ... ... like now ... ... just like now ... ... hold on to your power anchor so that it connects even more with you ... ... with your healing power ... ...

... ... [Continue the transition and let the client hold the healing anchor until hold the end of the session.] ... ...

#5

For Those Affected

... ... You know cancer well by now. You also know the difficult fight against ... ... you know that it helps you to stand up against it ... ... Sometimes you may also wish the sick ones to be able to simply let go of the cells of your body ... ... as if you could throw them overboard or spit out ... ... Then your thoughts circle around the question of why it hit you in particular ... ... Sometimes you might have thought that the illness was like a punishment ... ... Yes then again you realize that there are no such punishments ... ... All these probing thoughts burden you very much, perhaps more than you realize ... ... because you have so much to do with the disease do ... ... are constantly confronted with cancer, so that there is no other way than your thoughts to deal with it ... ... But today something else should happen ... ... Today it should be about to let go of all disturbing thoughts once ... ... these thoughts that tend to be slow in healing do ... ... As soon as you manage to let go of the disturbing thoughts, your organism can concentrate even better on the healing ... ... and you will feel more comfortable ... ... This requires that you change your thoughts and feelings ... ... So you want to Let go of those disturbing thoughts and feelings ... ... Maybe you are already excited to see how that works ... ... You imagine that every single thought is a small colored ball that is in your head ... ... All feelings are also located as small balls in your head ... ... so you just have to find the disturbing thoughts and feelings to let go of them ... ... you can recognize them by their color ... ... your breathing will help you ... ... For example, let's take a look at your depressed mood ... ... your tiredness and severity ... ... your inner depression ... ... So you can imagine that all thoughts and all feelings that belong to your depressed mood, the color blue ... ... [The colors can of course be exchanged; they are chosen arbitrarily and are filled with suggestions.] ... ... carry ... ... So there are a lot of little blue balls in your head that you can let go of ... ...You do this with your breathing ... ... you breathe in and the air you breathe flows through your head ... ... You can see it in your inner eye ... ... The air you breathe collects all blue thoughts and feelings and carry them with you ... ... And you breathe them out ... ... They come out of yours as soap bubbles nose and float through the room ... ... Lots of blue soap bubbles ... ... And one after the other dissolves ... ... they just burst ... ... and you carry on ... ... you inhale and collect all blue thoughts and feelings in ... ... you breathe them out like soap bubbles ... ... they float through the room and dissolve ... ... You repeat that with every breath. Your depressed mood is dissolving more and more ... ... You're deep inside is now leaving new thoughts arise ... ... You feel the feeling of hope ... ... It works by itself. You just keep breathing and watch the blue soap bubbles that ... ... Now let's look at your feelings of guilt ... ... because you have often accused yourself ... ... you may even now think that you did something wrong or that you were to blame and that's why you got sick ... ... All thoughts and feelings with guilt are connected are yellow ... ... So there are a lot of yellow balls in your head that you let go ... ... you breathe in and collect all the yellow thoughts and feelings ... ... and you breathe them out ... ... They come out of your nose as soap bubbles and float through the room ... ... Lots of yellow soap bubbles ... ... And one after the other dissolves ... ... They just burst ... ... And you go on ... ... you breathe in and collect all the yellow thoughts and feelings ... ... You breathe them out as soap bubbles ... ... They float through the room and dissolve ... ... That you repeat with every breath ... ... Your deep inner being lets new thoughts arise again. You become free and you realize that you are innocent ... ... It works by itself ... ... You just keep breathing and watch the yellow soap bubbles dissolve ... ... you are innocent ... ... you are and always will be innocent ... ... Next up is your perfectionism ... ... you know how it is ... ... you have so often tries to do everything particularly well ... ... to do everything better and better and not fail to have ... ... Also in the fight against your illness you gave everything again and again ... ... Perhaps there were times of desperation, but you kept pulling yourself up and moving on done ... ... All thoughts and feelings that deal with perfectionism or lead to perfectionism are red ... ... So there are a lot of red balls in your head that you let go of can ... ... you breathe in and collect all the red thoughts and feelings ... ... and you breathe them from ... ... They come out of your nose as soap bubbles and float through the room ... ... Louder red soap bubbles ... ... and one by one dissolves ... ... they just burst ... ... and you carry on ... ... you breathe in and collect all the red thoughts and feelings

... ... as soaps you breathe them out ... ... they float through the room and dissolve .. ... Repeat that with every breath ... ... your deep inner being lets new thoughts arise again. To the Instead of perfectionism comes serenity and consideration for yourself ... ... This is how by itself ... ... you just keep breathing and watch the red soap bubbles dissolve ... ... Serenity and consideration become stronger ... ... Serenity and consideration become stronger ... ...

... ... Your deep inner being impresses everything ... ... Deep down you know that you can actually breathe out all disturbing thoughts and feelings, today and every day in your life ... ... You also know that everything you let go of will be replaced by new, helping, constructive thoughts ... ... so you will freer and stronger ... ... so you have more strength for your recovery ... ... today you can you feel it ... ... So you can feel it every other day in your life ... ... whenever you want, you just close your eyes for a moment and breathe out everything that is disturbing as colored soap bubbles ... ... Just like today, they burst and dissolve ... ... just like today ... ... And you feel new strength ... ...

#6

For Those Affected

... ... You know what it's like to have a body that doesn't always work properly ... ... you know them days when it is not easy to get physically healthy ... ... And now you want that with everyone strength ... ...get physically healthy again ... ... as healthy as it can be ... ... as pain-free and flexible as possible ... ... Today you will find a helping hand deep inside you power ... ... a power that will help you to strengthen your body as much as possible... ... a force that can help you heal ... ... a force in you that can contribute to it can help you get well again ... ... as good as possible ... ... Maybe you know that yourself in difficult and even in seemingly hopeless situations, more is still possible than the mind can imagine ... ... more than the mind often wants to believe ... ... that's why you are here today ... ... because deep down you believe that everything is possible, what you imagine or you can simply wish ... ... To this end, you focus your mindfulness on the helping side today of your body, because there are also...... So today you are talking to your body...... you go into this direct contact and focus your mindfulness on everything that your body already has did for you when he was still healthy and many parts of your body are still ... ... you thank your body today for everything that has worked well until today ... ... Also for the fact that he can and will help you to become healthier ... ... First you address yourself to your hands. You say thank you that she always grabbed it have ... ... they have often held on ... ... often let go ... ... they do their vigorous service every day, as best they can ... ... they can also give you hints as to when it is better to let go should ... ... because when you let go your hands become free again and open to new things ... ... Eighth on the feeling in your hands ... ... they signal to you when you can also let go internally ... ... Also that which could make you sick or contributed to your illness ... ... Let get rid of it now and free yourself from it ... ... [what feels like a half-minute break] ... ... Then speak with your arms ... ... they hold your hands and lift loads ... ... you know how it is difficult to bear loads, internally and externally ... ... always have your arms with you helped ... ... you thank them now, and they will continue to help you ... ... because it is theirs task to lend a hand for you ... ... to access when opportunities arise ... ... to do that carry what you want to hold and finally let go of what you do with your hands you no longer need ... ... Next you turn to your back ... ... It carries a lot of burdens ...... It also keeps your body upright and straight ... ... Your back has been so often done good offices for you ... ... worked well all these years and never complained ... ... sometimes was he bent over from all the burden ... ... She pushed you down so that you couldn't follow could look in front ... ... but your back has always helped you to straighten up to be able to look forward again ... ... and to go on powerfully ... ... you thank your back today for his faithful service that he has done all these years until today ... ... Then speak you with the internal organs ... ... you thank them for having done their work so well so often ... ... the interaction of all organs makes life possible. And every organ has always tries to make the best possible contribution ... ... every healthy thing still does it today and even organs that have become sick continue to work for us ... ... as best they can ... ... they work like a chain and pull together ...

... ... But sometimes a chain breaks or can no longer work as hard because a chain link has become weaker ... ... but all of them other organs try to keep the internal functioning of the organism upright ... ... they do the same weakens out as best they can ... ... Your organs have also been doing this for many years ... ... until today they do it ... ... Then you direct yourself to your heart ... ... It keeps pumping blood into it body and supplies all organs with oxygen and life ... ... It brings the oxygen and all that nutrients in the blood in all muscles like fuel in an engine ... ... It keeps beating ... ... every second of your life ... ... day and night ... ... you thank your heart that it all has struck the years for you, without a break ... ... in quiet, but also in stormy moments ... ... It always works and only rests in the small breaks between the beats ... ... yours source of life ... ... You then focus your mindfulness on your legs ... ... You say thank you to them for carrying your body for so long ... ... they carry the body, hold it upright and take you from one place to another ... ... they can move you, but can also stop to pause and linger, because that is also important and necessary ... ... but you also helped to be faster ... ... to overtake ... ... they accompany you faithfully and to help ... ... companions in the truest sense of the word ... ... After all, you address yourself to your skin ... ... Today you thank your skin ... ...

for it, that she gave you protection and warmth ... ... for protecting the bones and the insides from attack ... ... for taking up dirt and washing it off again, so that your insides remain clean and clear ... ...

... ... Now turn to the sick spot or the sick area of your body ... ... concentrate focus on the diseased organ or the diseased area of your body ... ... remember how long too this area of your body was healthy and try to say thank you for the time as your whole body was still healthy ... ... You will succeed, because you know that it will help you find your peace to do with your body ... ... Now you allow yourself some rest ... ... You let your body rest and trust in its help...... You also tell your body to help...... you makes a pact with all your body parts ... ... you assure your body that you will take care of it carefully and that it will always have rest to recover from the rigors of treatment you give ... ... in return, your body tries to become healthier and stronger as quickly as possible ... ... that should be your pact ... ...

#7

For Those Affected

The following hypnosis session works with the classic arm levitation (floating arm). With the help of suggestions or images, the arm levitation gives the impression that the body of the client can be moved without his involvement. The required muscle contraction is performed unconsciously, expressed somewhat imprecisely but understandably: the subconscious the client makes the movement that appears to the client to be controlled by others. Levitations increase belief in the special effects of hypnosis and show the client that it is gives more than what he actively decides and can consciously and deliberately influence. It is important that the client can observe the floating and then cataleptically (rigid) arm himself with his or her eyes. So always leave that with arm levitations and catalepsies open your eyes to see the result. Many clients otherwise believe that the entire Arm movement was just an illusion, some feel the movement when closed Eyes not very clear either. Don't worry, when you open your eyes you won't lose your trance and your catalepsy will remain stable! The stronger a sick person's own belief in them the more positive the treatment progress is, the more self-healing power of his organism is Cancer as well as all other diseases. Of course, hypnosis is not a miracle. So never promise a certain success (by the way, this is forbidden for all therapists anyway).

... ... I will now help you to really activate your own self-healing power ... ... it can help you help make the most significant progress possible in recovery ... ... We will today strengthen the self-healing power of your organism together ... ...

... ... [Now follows arm levitation, for which there are numerous possibilities. You will be the following not being able to read the text easily. At least you should go to the next section "Catalepsy" skips over when the arm has already risen far up so that the elbow is away from the Underlay takes off. If the proposed text is not sufficient, extend it or repeat it him until the arm goes up. If you put persuasiveness and emphasis in your voice, it will be quite easy.] ... ...

Levitation phase

... ... Take a look at your right arm and imagine that a big red balloon is tied to it ... ... with a string around your wrist ... ... The balloon is filled with a very light gas, so that it rises ... ... The balloon rises into the air and pulls your arm up with it ... ... Imagine this huge red balloon and watch it go ... ... it rises higher and higher and pulls your arm up ... ... Your arm follows the balloon and rises higher and higher ... ... your arm becomes light as a feather and just rises up ... ... leave it just happen and be happy about it ... ... A huge red balloon takes your arm with it up ... ... Your arm rises higher and higher ... ... It gets lighter and lighter and rises into the air ... ... Your arm rises higher and higher ... ... higher and higher ... ... just like that ... ... just like that ... ... outstanding ... ... your arm is light as a feather and rises all by itself, all by itself ... ... So it's easy ... ... Your arm rises higher and higher ... ... higher and higher ... ... Look at the balloon afterwards ... ... the balloon rises in the air and pulls your arm with it ... ... it pulls and pulls ... ... he pulls and pulls on your arm ... ... pulls and pulls ... ...

atalepsy phase

...... And now your arm becomes completely rigid and firm ...... [emphasis on the voice] ...... your arm becomes held exactly like that, it stays in exactly this position ...... your arm is light as a feather and absolutely firm ...... He is immobile ...... absolutely immobile ...... Nothing and nobody can hold your arm now still move ...... it remains rigid and firm and light as a feather ...... as firm as an iron bar ...... just like that ...... that's right ...... you can even look at your arm, you can look at it, he remains in exactly this position ...... Now open your eyes and look at your arm, the remains in exactly this position ...... now! ...... [If the eyes are not opened, please help a little. Consists in a deep trance little motivation to open their eyes, and it is also difficult for the client because he is very is tired. Help something like this ... You can open your eyes, you can. So go ahead, open your eyes now and look at your arm! ...] ...... Now close your eyes again and sink into a deep trance ...... Your subconscious becomes you help now, it has already helped you because it has raised your arm for you and is now holding it still firm ...... Now your subconscious will help you, your self-healing power to make you stronger and to make as much of it available to you as possible ...... your arm will immediately flexible again and your subconscious provides you with the greatest possible self-healing power ... ...

Consolidation (post-hypnotic assignment)

... ... Your arm is now flexible again and sinks very slowly onto the surface, your subconscious activates your self-healing power ... ... Your arm now slowly sinks back down ... ... very slowly ... ... and as soon as it arrives on the mat, you have self-healing power your organism is fully available ... ... This activation only lasts as long as yours arm needed to reach the surface ... ... Your arm sinks down at exactly the speed that your subconscious needs to optimally increase your self-healing power and to make it available to you ... ... and as soon as he touches the surface, your self-healing power is fully available and helps you with your recovery ... ... your arm slowly sinks onto the seat ... ...

... ... [Keep on making suggestions until the arm reaches the surface. Then please solve ide motor / catalepsy with the following suggestion on] ... ...

… … Your arm is now completely mobile and under your control. Move your arm and your hand and check that you actually have full control over your body

#8

For Those Affected

... ... You have dealt extensively with all the things that can have contributed to your illness ... ... it there were physical reasons for it and physical conditions ... ... but you also know that there are psychological conditions that contribute to your illness ... ... how it works, how well yours The prognosis can be ... ... You have long since realized that your illness has a very high proportion psychological factors mean that you have to deal with your thoughts and feelings if you not only get healthy, but also stay healthy in the long term want ... ... and that's exactly what you want ... ... get healthy and then stay healthy ... ... you want it more than ever before ... ... get healthy and stay healthy ... ... So now concentrate on the area or part of your body that is affected by the disease most affected is...... Put all your attention on this area as if it were there just this one part of your body ... ... if you want, you can look at your body from the outside, as if you were standing next to you and could look at your body ... ... take this Now focus entirely on the area or area of your body affected by the disease your attention ... ... and give yourself mindfulness and care ... ... mindfulness and care ... ... Perhaps you are also wondering how that works, yourself or your body To be mindful ... ... It's very simple ... ... Just be there ... ... Just think of yours Body and stay with your thoughts with him ... ... Nothing else is important now ... ... That is enough ... ... Mindfulness is loving attention to the thoughts ... ... and that is very much more than we usually have left for ourselves ... ... we often turn to others, that do you know well ... ... so now turn to yourself and give yourself attention and loving thoughts ... ... Go with all your conscious thoughts to the place of your illness and feel there into it ... ... direct all of your mindfulness there ... ... Imagine a red dot on yours Body in front of the sick spot ... ... as if this spot was marked so that you can always put it in the Can take a look ... ... feel into your body, at precisely this point and sink into this point of your body ... ... dive with your attention there ... ... always leave it get darker ... ... sink in deeper and deeper ... ... ever deeper and deeper ... ... it gets darker and darker ... ... your thoughts get quieter and slowly fade into the background ... ... your thoughts fade into the background, because now comes it just depends on your feeling ... ... that feeling that sits so deep in your body, at the point of your illness ... ... much deeper than the body can feel ... ... very deep in the emotions ... behind the sick part of your body you will find a special feeling that is now becoming increasingly clear will...... let this feeling become conscious, however it may be...... however it is may feel ... ... It is the feeling that is behind and in your illness. This feeling you can now clearly see ... ... Do not judge it, because feelings are neither good nor bad ...... Feelings are an expression of our inner experiences and experiences...... of ours reactions to our living conditions and events ... ... Exactly this feeling, that behind the red dot is now becoming increasingly clear, can help you to get well again ... ... Exactly this feeling can help you to free yourself from thoughts that make you sick, so that your organism gets stronger for your recovery ... ... you let the feeling go ... ... you just let it become conscious so that you can decouple it from the illness ... ... you can also feel the feeling even without illness ... You can feel this feeling now ... ... and you can let it become clearer ... ... clearer ... ... more consciously ... ... let it become very intense, however it may be may feel ... ... It did not cause your illness, but it did contribute to it ... ... It slows down the healing ... ... But today everything will be different ... ... Today you recognize the feeling ... ... Today you free it and thus uncouple it from you and an illness ... ... It is as if you would open an inner window from which the feeling can now escape ... ... This is how you free yours illness from this feeling ... ... Your body can heal much better now because this feeling is it has now become clear to you ... ... but even if you are not yet sure what feeling it actually is ... ... if you are can't feel it so clearly now ... ... so you know that there is a feeling behind the illness that is now in motion ... ... The feeling is in motion and can now be slowly dissolved ... ... like a warm air stream it can escape through the window inside you ... ... simply dissolve into thin air, because you now know that this feeling exists or gives a feeling that can now be resolved ... ... You no longer need it, because it has long belonged to the Past of ... ... Now the feeling of the illness is released ... ... now disconnected ... ... Now! ... ...

... ... This will make you much more free inside ... ... maybe you can feel it because you can breathe better or you just feel lighter inside ... ... the healing can actually go faster now ... ... really amazing how quickly your body can recover after the deep lying feelings get in motion and be replaced … … this is exactly what is happening … … detachment … … exactly that … … detachment … … Whenever you concentrate on your body, exactly on that place that should heal again, you give yourself mindfulness and concentrate on this place … … So you can strengthen your life force yourself, strengthen your courage, strengthen your hope and also your confidence … … so you can experience healing … …

#9

For Those Affected

... ... You have been through a lot lately, taking on the stress of chemotherapy because you decided to go this route of treatment ... ... At the same time you go a way of healing, which is also an inner way ... ... because deep within you lies the power that you need to get through this time and to recover again and again, between the chemotherapy treatments and after the last session, so that you can then fully recover ... Breathe deeply in and out and relax your muscles ... ... your body comes to rest, as if you want to fall asleep to dream a beautiful dream ... ... deep in your imagination ... ... you pose embark on an inner journey ... ... a journey to a faraway country that is also very close ...... The land of your dreams...... Feel the rhythm of your breathing and follow it...... with the wind of your breath you leave your thoughts and go to the land of dreams ... ... You are sitting in a meadow that has dried up completely ... ... The grass is yellow, almost brown and everything looks very dreary ... ... you look around, but everything is so dry here, so drained ... ... Then you notice that you are sitting on the bank of a river ... ... But the river bed has no water more ... ... The power of the river seems to succumb and the meadow that was once there is blooming Life seems interrupted ... ... Life seems to stand still ... ... You close your eyes and feel your breath ... ... you can hear your breath clearly ... ... and in the same rhythm your breath also blows the wind gently through the land of dreams ... ... you hear the gentle rustling of the wind, which you can soon no longer distinguish from the sound of your breath ... ... The sound of your breathing and the wind merge into one another ... ... That is breathing and wind same ... ... exactly the same ... ... And if you focus your attention and all your mindfulness on the sound of the wind, you will hear a soft whisper in the wind ... ... a tender voice that speaks to you ... ... the wind whispers to you: Everything should bloom ... ... Everything should bloom ... ... Don't wish it ... ... don't long for it come over ... ... and then the wind whispers: Just imagine ... ... get an idea of it, that's enough ... ... And so you follow the words of the wind and imagine how everything will bloom and will find its way back to the old beauty and splendor ... ... You imagine how beautiful this one meadow will look like, with lots of flowers and green grass, maybe with friendly animals ... ... with trees that bear sweet fruit ... ... Then you hear the whispering of the wind that tells you: So is it right ... ... That's good ... ... Then you let the picture in your inner eye become clearer ... ... For so long you have only dealt with the fact that the cancer has grown in you ... ... that this disease has spread as if it had been fertilized ... ... But diseases are sometimes there, and we cannot understand why this is happening ... ... We look for explanations and don't find an answer ... ... Then it's time we focused again on what should really grow in us ... ... life should grow ... ... health should grow ... ... hope and joy should grow ... ... because that is exactly what makes our inner world lively and colorful ... ... that is exactly what makes the meadows and fields bloom deep within us ... ... and suddenly you hear rushing water ... ... You open your eyes and look around ... ...water flows through the river bed again ... ... It fills with bubbling water, which afterwards life feels ... ... for progress ... ... for fresh energy ... ... It tears the dry dust of the river bed with itself and turns dark ... ... it's still cloudy, because all the dust and dirt that has accumulated, must first be washed away ... ... But gradually the water becomes clearer and clearer ... ... because life returns ... ... the dust of heavy thoughts and Fears will be washed away ... ... The water gets cleaner and clearer until it finally comes crystal clear and flowing through the river bed ... ... you can see all the way to the bottom ... ... to very deep into the river bed ... ... you can see every stone on the ground ... ... pure, fresh Water ... ... so clear that you can look right down to the bottom of the river bed, very deep down ... ... a beautiful river arises as if by itself ... ... Then you look across the meadow and suddenly small green shoots appear everywhere, emerging from the soil grow so fast that you can watch ... ... grass starts to close before your eyes grow ... ... The meadow suddenly turns green again and everything looks new ... ... It starts to bloom ... ... blooming flowers appear within seconds, nourished by the fresh water of the river in the land of dreams ... ... And so it goes on around you and deep inside you ... ... power blooms ... ... you bloom yourself again ... ... trees suddenly appear on the beautiful meadow, that bear ripe fruit ... ... As in a time lapse, you can watch the watching plants and enjoying them ... ... all of this happens because it is your imagination, because you created a picture of it and put it in front of you looked at your inner eye without expectation ... ... life is back ... ... and also your strength will increase again ... ... You close your eyes and take your body very clearly and consciously true ... ...

... ... You feel that this river of life flows deep inside you and brings new life ...... strength and patience for the upcoming challenges and always new blossoming of your life ... ... You think about the fact that the land of dreams is deep inside you. There was it always. I'm just telling you about it ... ...

#10

For those who are preparing for the approaching death

...... You go to the land of dreams ...... You stand on a blooming meadow and look into the distance ...... You can see the entire dreamland; look into a wide valley ...... And you stand up in the sun ...... you are here to make your peace ...... also for yourself to say goodbye, because your time here on earth is coming to an end ...... You know it, and you are introducing yourself very consciously and actively ...... here and today, at this very moment ...... But before you leave this world, you want to make your peace ... ... with unresolved situations ...... maybe with certain people ...... you can do today what you still want to clean or lock ...... maybe that is no longer possible in your waking world, but here in the land of dreams it can happen ...... dream and reality are only one breath apart ...... Everything that happens here in the land of dreams happens whole deep in your heart and is reality ...... your reality, and only that counts ...... only on it depends ...... so you go and do this Easter march in the valley of silence ...... you go down over five large levels into this valley, in which everything is quiet and peaceful ... ... on everyone Level you make peace, if you want it that way ... ... decide for yourself, it is your truth ... ... Your march for peace begins on the fifth level ... ... You look up at the sky and see a message there in bold letters between the clouds. It says: do yours peace now and get free! ... ... Then you come to level four and meet a group of children who play and hardly notice that you are there ... ... One of the children looks the same how you looked when you were a child ... ... it's you yourself, you meet yourself here in one other time, in your childhood ... ... As a visitor to your past, images of earlier times arise around you ... ... a scene is built up that shows you where or with whom in yours childhood you still want to make your peace ... ... Look at the pictures in peace, leave them simply arise and be there, whatever you see, feel or experience ... ... maybe became much has already been cleared up or clarified, and it is possible that much of what happened once remains is, stand like this and can no longer be changed ... ... But you can make your peace now, if you want to ... ... Maybe you want to say something to a person or you just want to be there ... ... do it the way it is right for you, just follow your feeling ... ... take your time until you hear my voice again ... ... [please give what feels like a minute, then continue] ... ... Now prepare yourself to continue your Easter march ... ... You go on to the plain three and you arrive in your youth ... ... Here, too, pictures and scenes from that time are created but above all, there are very special events ... ... the events that show you where and with whom you can still make your peace ... ... Take a look at the events and pictures, what however you see or experience ... ... Here too there may be difficult situations, maybe events that have remained open forever ... ... Today you can end them deep in your heart ... ... You can make your peace now, if you want to ... ... Maybe you want to say something to a person or you just want to be there ... ... do it the way it is right for you, just follow your feeling ... ... take your time until you hear my voice again ... ... [a felt one Please give a minute, then continue] ... ... Now prepare yourself to continue your Easter march ... ... You go on, deeper and deeper into the valley of silence and come to level two... ... that is the level of your adult life ... ... Here you can find everything again, what you have already lived through as an adult ... ... you can recognize situations, meet people who mean something to you or who have played a major role in your life ... ... some helpful and constructive, others with anger and injustice ... ... Whom or whatever you are meet here, it is right, because you can see where you have not yet made peace ... ... Today you can do it ... ... You can make your peace now, if you want to ... ... Maybe you want to say something to a person or you just want to be there ... ... Do it like this, how it is right for you, just follow your feeling ... ... take your time until you hear my voice like that ... ... [please give what feels like a minute, then continue] ... ... prepare yourself now before to continue your Easter march ... ... You go further into the deep valley and come to one on the level ... ... Here you meet the person who is most important to you in life ... ... Possibly there is nothing unexplained with this person ... ... maybe everything has been discussed and everything is understood between you ... ... but maybe there is still something uncleaned here and there ... ... You can either make your peace with everything that is still open with this dear person is or with everything that could possibly be open without your knowing it ... ... But even if everything is already in order ... ... you can make your peace together ... ... make peace with her illness ... ...

peace with fate ... ... peace with God, if you can believe in him, or just peace with another authority in which you can believe ... ... you can now yours make peace, if you want it that way ... ... Maybe you want to say something to a person or you want to say something to God ... ... do it the way it is right for you, just follow your feeling ... ... take your time until you hear my voice again ... ... [please give what feels like a minute, then continue] ... ... Now prepare to continue your Easter march ... ... Finally you go all the way through the valley of silence and meet yourself at the end of the valley ... ... you meet yourself like a twin sister / brother and make peace with yourself now ... ... You forgive yourself for everything you have ever accused yourself of ... ... You treat yourself with respect and dignity and thank yourself for everything you have tried in your life, for all that you have succeeded in and also for what you have not succeeded, because you have yours Humanity shown ... ... Make your peace with yourself now ... ... Do it as it is for you is correct, just follow your feeling ... ... take your time until you hear my voice again ... ... [Please give what feels like a minute, then continue] ... ...

Distribution, publication, and copying in any form are prohibited and subject to damages.

Overview of All Titles in the Series "Ten Hypnoses"

Volume 1: Smoking Cessation
Volume 2: Anxiety and Restlessness
Volume 3: Burnout
Volume 4: Reducing Overweight
Volume 5: Coping with the Past
Volume 6: Suicidal Thoughts and Attempts
Volume 7: Psycho-Oncology
Volume 8: Obsessions and Tics
Volume 9: Self-Confidence and Decision-Making
Volume 10: Grief Work
Volume 11: Psychosomatics
Volume 12: Chronic Pain
Volume 13: Depressive Thoughts
Volume 14: Panic Attacks
Volume 15: Domestic Violence, Victim Support
Volume 16: Post-Traumatic Stress
Volume 17: Exam Anxiety and Stage Fright
Volume 18: Anti-Violence Training, Offender Support
Volume 19: Addiction Tendencies
Volume 20: Social Phobia and Fear of Contact
Volume 21: Nail Biting
Volume 22: Self-Awareness and Self-Love
Volume 23: Teeth Grinding and Night Clenching
Volume 24: Feelings of Guilt
Volume 25: Fear in Crowds
Volume 26: Fear of Flying, Aviophobia
Volume 27: Fear in Enclosed Spaces, Claustrophobia
Volume 28: Tinnitus, Ear Noises
Volume 29: Fear of Heights
Volume 30: Neurodermatitis

Copying, publishing, and sharing with third parties are only permitted with the written consent of the author. Please observe the notes on copyright and usage.

Volume 31: Finding Inner Balance
Volume 32: Overcoming Loneliness
Volume 33: Fear of Illness, Hypochondria
Volume 34: Anticipatory Anxiety, Fear of Fear
Volume 35: Jealousy in Relationships
Volume 36: Driving Anxiety
Volume 37: New Start after Separation
Volume 38: Fear of Injections
Volume 39: Heart Anxiety Neurosis
Volume 40: Overcoming Resentment and Anger
Volume 41: Resolving Blockages and Positive Thinking
Volume 42: Stress Reduction, Stress Management
Volume 43: Body Relaxation
Volume 44: Deep Relaxation
Volume 45: Fear of the Dark
Volume 46: Falling Asleep and Staying Asleep
Volume 47: Compulsive Buying
Volume 48: Restless Legs Syndrome
Volume 49: Bulimia
Volume 50: Anorexia
Volume 51: Overcoming Nightmares
Volume 52: Imagined Deformity
Volume 53: Overcoming Distrust, Finding Trust
Volume 54: Processing Failures
Volume 55: Humiliation, Emotional Hurt
Volume 56: Distressing Compassion, Vicarious Suffering
Volume 57: Self-Forgiveness
Volume 58: Self-Awareness, Self-Confidence
Volume 59: Saying No
Volume 60: Assertiveness
Volume 61: Setting Boundaries and Self-Assertion
Volume 62: Decision-Making Ability

Volume 63: Success Orientation
Volume 64: Ruminating, Circular Thinking
Volume 65: Accepting Pregnancy
Volume 66: Birth Preparation
Volume 67: Spiritual Opening
Volume 68: Joy of Life and Inner Lightness
Volume 69: Patience and Inner Peace
Volume 70: Fibromyalgia and Rheumatism
Volume 71: Irritable Bowel Syndrome, Crohn's Disease
Volume 72: Fear of Nausea, Emetophobia
Volume 73: Stuttering and Cluttering, Speech Flow Disorders
Volume 74: Concentration and Knowledge Anchoring
Volume 75: Vitality and Spontaneity
Volume 76: Searching for Meaning and Finding Goals
Volume 77: Life Crises, Life Events
Volume 78: Workaholism, Goal Obsession
Volume 79: Helper Syndrome, Helpless Helpers
Volume 80: Medication Abuse
Volume 81: Gambling Addiction
Volume 82: Internet Addiction, Smartphone Addiction
Volume 83: Hoarding Disorder, Compulsive Collecting
Volume 84: Conspiracy Thoughts, Overvalued Ideas
Volume 85: Fear of Operations and Treatments
Volume 86: Fear of Aging
Volume 87: Travel Anxiety
Volume 88: Anxiety When Urinating, Paruresis
Volume 89: Fear of Intimacy and Togetherness
Volume 90: Fear of Blushing
Volume 91: Coming Out in Homosexuality
Volume 92: Charisma Training
Volume 93: Migraines and Chronic Headaches
Volume 94: Overcoming Allergies, Bronchial Asthma

Volume 95: Normalizing Blood Pressure
Volume 96: Compulsive Perfectionism
Volume 97: Sports Hypnosis, Motivation
Volume 98: Sports Hypnosis, Performance Enhancement
Volume 99: Determination and Focus
Volume 100: Encountering the Inner Child
Volume 101: Cravings, Binge Eating
Volume 102: Stimulating Metabolism
Volume 103: Bipolar Mood Swings
Volume 104: Borderline, Identity Crises
Volume 105: Hypomania, Euphoria, Mania
Volume 106: Restlessness, Agitation
Volume 107: Nervous Breakdown
Volume 108: Adjustment Disorders
Volume 109: Self-Alienation, Depersonalization
Volume 110: Ending Self-Pity
Volume 111: Primary Gain of Illness
Volume 112: Secondary Gain of Illness
Volume 113: Bullying, Victim Support
Volume 114: Letting Go of Envy and Jealousy
Volume 115: Fear of Spiders, Arachnophobia
Volume 116: Fear of Dogs or Cats
Volume 117: Fear of Strangers, Xenophobia
Volume 118: Excessive Worries, Generalized Anxiety
Volume 119: Strengthening Sense of Responsibility
Volume 120: Unrequited Love, Heartache
Volume 121: Work-Life Balance
Volume 122: Letting Go of Unattainable Goals
Volume 123: Allowing and Accepting Help
Volume 124: Letting Go of Adult Children
Volume 125: Tourette Syndrome
Volume 126: Life Changes and New Starts

Volume 127: Accepting Life in a Wheelchair
Volume 128: Understanding and Overcoming Homesickness
Volume 129: Understanding and Overcoming Wanderlust
Volume 130: Dizziness, Meniere's Disease
Volume 131: Overcoming Aggression
Volume 132: Cutting and Self-Harm
Volume 133: Hair Pulling, Trichotillomania
Volume 134: Postpartum Depression
Volume 135: For Relatives of Dementia Patients
Volume 136: Self-Harm, Artificial Disorders
Volume 137: Activating Self-Healing Powers
Volume 138: Preventing Depression Relapse
Volume 139: Reactive Psychoses, Follow-Up
Volume 140: Obsessive Thoughts and Impulses
Volume 141: Compulsive Checking
Volume 142: Compulsive Counting, Symmetry Obsession
Volume 143: Compulsive Washing, Cleanliness Obsession
Volume 144: Compulsive Questioning
Volume 145: Dissociative Paralysis
Volume 146: Phantom Pain
Volume 147: Overcoming Complaining
Volume 148: Hay Fever, Pollen Allergy
Volume 149: Sexual Abuse, Victim Support
Volume 150: Standing Strong Against Sexism, #metoo
Volume 151: Binge Eating
Volume 152: Overcoming Thoughts of Revenge
Volume 153: Detachment from the Aggressor, Stockholm Syndrome
Volume 154: Courage to Separate
Volume 155: Chronic Fatigue, Exhaustion
Volume 156: Fear of the Future, Existential Anxiety
Volume 157: Excessive Worry About Children
Volume 158: Fear of Failure

Volume 159: Ending Distrust and Control
Volume 160: Dejection, Dysphoria
Volume 161: Boreout, Chronic Boredom
Volume 162: Bipolar Disorders, Relapse Prevention
Volume 163: Mania, Relapse Prevention
Volume 164: Nihilism, Feelings of Worthlessness
Volume 165: Thumb Sucking
Volume 166: Being Brave
Volume 167: Being Proud
Volume 168: Overcoming Shyness
Volume 169: Being Able to Delegate Responsibility
Volume 170: Being Able to Show Emotions
Volume 171: Letting Go of Guilt, Victim Support
Volume 172: Processing Guilt, Offender Support
Volume 173: Mood Swings, Cyclothymia
Volume 174: Lack of Drive, Vital Sadness
Volume 175: Hearing Voices with Reality Reference
Volume 176: Confident Communication
Volume 177: Standing Up for Oneself
Volume 178: Taking New Paths
Volume 179: Confident Job Application
Volume 180: No Longer Being Taken Advantage Of
Volume 181: End of Submissiveness
Volume 182: Depressive Numbness
Volume 183: Mood Drops, Affective Incontinence
Volume 184: Mood Instability
Volume 185: Somatoform Disorders
Volume 186: Stomach Ulcer, Psychosomatic
Volume 187: Accepting Amputation
Volume 188: Overcoming and Letting Go of Hatred
Volume 189: Ending Accusations
Volume 190: Allowing Tears, Being Able to Cry

Volume 191: Finding and Sorting Repressed Feelings
Volume 192: Somatoform Pain
Volume 193: Living Autonomously
Volume 194: Anhedonia, Joylessness
Volume 195: Persistent Sadness
Volume 196: Obesity, Food Addiction
Volume 197: Parents of Abused Children
Volume 198: Letting Go and Letting Be
Volume 199: Childhood Sexual Abuse
Volume 200: Fear of Loss

www.ingramcontent.com/pod-product-compliance
Lightning Source LLC
Chambersburg PA
CBHW030456220526
45464CB00006B/2556